HASHIMOTO'S THYROIDITIS
SMASHED!

**The Ultimate Guide To Overcoming
Hashimoto's Thyroiditis Disease**

HASHIMOTO'S DIET

HYPOTHYROIDISM, HYPERTHYROIDISM,

THYROIDITIS

Second Edition

BLAKE NICOLE

© 2015

COPYRIGHT NOTICE

DISCLAIMER

This book is not intended as a substitute for the medical advice of physicians. The reader should regularly consult a physician in matters relating to his/her health and particularly with respect to any symptoms that may require diagnosis or medical attention.

CONTENTS

INTRODUCTION

You are probably reading this book because you or someone you know has been diagnosed with Hashimoto's Thyroiditis Disease. You probably have many questions about this disease and how you can best deal with it. You may wonder how much this is going to change your life and if you will ever again be able to enjoy life with this debilitating disease.

This book will attempt to answer those questions, as well as explaining what Hashimoto's Thyroiditis is exactly, how it affects the body, what the causes and symptoms are and what you can do to help alleviate the effects of this disease.

We will first learn a little about the history of this disease, when it was discovered and why it was often misdiagnosed as other diseases, causing patients to be unresponsive to treatments and leading to much pain, and even death. Thanks to Hashimoto's discovery of this disease, doctors are now able to diagnose and properly treat this, improving hundreds of thousands of people's lives.

We will also learn about one of the major effects of Hashimoto's disease, which is a condition known as Hypothyroidism. You will learn what hypothyroidism is, how it is treated, and most importantly, you will learn how to live with this condition so that it need not be a debilitating illness.

Many people who suffer from this illness have come to believe that Hashimoto's thyroiditis is a life sentence, and that they will never be able to live a normal life. They feel that they are doomed to a life of gaining unwanted pounds, and that there is very little they can do to change this condition, due to the general effects of the disease. However, this book's aim is to help you to get rid of these preconceptions and show you that there really can be a long and healthy life after being diagnosed with Hashimoto's Thyroiditis.

You will learn about the proper foods to eat in order to maintain a healthy weight, even with the effects of hypothyroidism, and we will also touch on how you can take control of your lifestyle, in order to effectively combat Hashimoto's Thyroiditis and overcome the effects of the disease. In addition, we'll be going over the foods you'll need to avoid, foods that can actually contribute to the troubling effects of the disease and make things worse.

By the time you are finished reading this book, we believe that you will see that this disease need not be a defeating life sentence, but can be the start of a whole new healthy lifestyle. We feel sure that you'll learn that you can not only overcome this disease, but you can take the proper steps to change your lifestyle—one step at a time—so that you may become even healthier, have even more energy and vitality than you had, before you or your loved one was diagnosed with this awful illness.

You do not need to submit yourself to this disease, and you should not allow yourself to become discouraged by this diagnosis. You can choose instead to consider this diagnosis to be an opportunity to re-examine your lifestyle and your choices, an opportunity to enable you to overcome the disease and excel in your life. You will always have Hashimoto's Thyroiditis, but you don't have to let it defeat you. You can overcome it and be even stronger and better than you were before you ever even heard of it.

Let's get started, shall we?

A BRIEF HISTORY OF HASHIMOTO'S THYROIDITIS DISEASE

Before 1912, many people were suffering from an unknown disease that was often misdiagnosed as depression, chronic fatigue syndrome or even fibromyalgia. As the doctors tried to treat the patients, far too many of them inevitably failed to respond to their treatments, often suffering from hypothyroidism symptoms that would mysteriously change to hyperthyroidism, and then back again. Thousands of doctors were quite perplexed by these odd changes, and would often try treatments for many different diseases, almost always to no avail.

Then one day, in 1912, a Japanese Doctor named Hashimoto Hakaru described a new autoimmune disease, in which the thyroid gland is gradually attacked and destroyed by the immune system. This, finally, explained why someone can have an extreme excess of thyroid hormones in their system one day (hyperthyroidism), and far too little the next day (hypothyroidism). Doctors were finally able to pinpoint and treat this disease with a great deal of success, now that it was possible to have it properly diagnosed.

The actual name for this autoimmune disease is Chronic Lymphocytic Thyroiditis, but it is far more commonly known today as Hashimoto's Thyroiditis or Hashimoto's Disease, in honor of the doctor who first identified it. The disease was, and is still today, far too often misdiagnosed by doctors, but with the knowledge of this treatable disease that has been added to the physician's arsenal of information over the last hundred years, as doctors became more aware of the proper tests and symptoms, more patients have been properly diagnosed and treated.

While Hashimoto's Disease is still misdiagnosed many times today, a vast number of cases are caught and treated with much more success, and so thousands of people have been able to combat this disease and live normal lives. If left untreated, however, the disease can cause muscle failure, and even heart failure in some cases. Children with Hashimoto's thyroiditis can have their growth disrupted if it's left undiagnosed and untreated, possibly even to the point where they may require growth hormone therapy.

A simple test for thyroid antibodies (or anti-thyroid peroxidase antibodies) in the blood stream is usually all that is necessary to properly diagnose this disease; however, seronegative thyroiditis is also possible, in which there are no circulating autoantibodies.

Once properly diagnosed, the disease can be treated with thyroid hormone replacement therapy, which can be synthetic or can be produced from animals. The thyroid treatment does not cure the disease, and unfortunately, the patient must continue to take hormone replacements throughout their lives. However, this is as easy as taking a pill every day.

The most common symptoms of Hashimoto's are:

- Constipation
- Depression
- Fatigue and muscle weakness
- High Cholesterol
- Migraines
- Sensitivity to heat and cold
- Weight gain

Having one or more of these symptoms doesn't necessarily indicate Hashimoto's thyroiditis, but when you see that several symptoms are combined, it's a good idea to see your doctor and ask to have your thyroid checked, just to be sure. Many doctors still misdiagnose this, as they look at individual symptoms as indications of other possible diseases or disorders, and may not initiate the proper tests; however, more doctors today are aware of this debilitating illness and do check the thyroid as part of a regular screening. If you or someone you know might be suffering from more than two or three of these symptoms, it would be a very good idea to see the doctor, and to be sure that he or she has performed a thyroid test.

HASHIMOTO'S DISEASE & HYPOTHYROIDISM

There are many who confuse Hashimoto's Disease with Hypothyroidism. The thing to remember is that Hashimoto's Disease (or Hashimoto's thyroiditis, autoimmune thyroiditis, or chronic lymphocytic thyroiditis) is a disease, whereas Hypothyroidism is a condition commonly caused by Hashimoto's Disease.

First, let's look at what the thyroid gland is. The thyroid gland shaped like a butterfly and is positioned just in front of the windpipe or trachea, partially surrounding it, and just under what we know as the voice box, which is actually called the larynx. The thyroid gland utilizes iodine from the foods we eat to make the two essential thyroid hormones that control the way our bodies make use of the energy we obtain from the nutrients we consume.

The parathyroid glands are four very small additional glands which are located slightly behind the thyroid itself. These glands produce a substance called parathyroid hormone that helps to regulate the volume of calcium and phosphorous in your bloodstream. The parathyroid glands are also very important, and can be involved in the problems which lead to hypothyroidism and/or Hashimoto's Thyroiditis.

Hypothyroidism is the condition in which the body does not have sufficient thyroid hormone. Without sufficient thyroid hormone, the body is unable to metabolize energy from foods normally, which causes the symptoms associated with a slow metabolism. It is estimated that approximately 10 million Americans suffer from hypothyroidism, with a large percentage of them not even being aware that they have it.

The two most common causes of hypothyroidism are 1

The most common cause, however, is still Hashimoto's thyroiditis, which is also a form of thyroid inflammation, but is caused by the body's own immune system.

There are other, less common causes of hypothyroidism, such as when the normal or healthy thyroid gland is not making enough thyroid hormone due to problems in the pituitary gland. If the pituitary does not produce enough TSH (thyroid stimulating hormone) the thyroid can't produce enough of its own hormone simply because it hasn't received the proper signal to start producing it.

In addition, certain conditions in the hypothalamus can cause the problem, by failing to produce a hormone called TRH (thyrotropin releasing hormone), which tells the pituitary gland to produce TSH.

Sometimes, certain thyroid conditions require the surgical removal of part or all of the thyroid, and if the body doesn't have enough cells left in the body after this surgery then the patient will develop hypothyroidism. This is often the goal in patients suffering from thyroid cancer. If, however, only part of the thyroid is removed, as happens in many cases, the remaining part may still be capable of producing enough hormone to meet the needs of the body, and make it possible to live normally without hormone supplements. Your doctor will determine whether additional medications or hormonal supplements are necessary if you are one of those who fit into this small category.

Symptoms of hypothyroidism include (but are not limited to):

- o Abnormal menstrual cycles
- o Constipation
- o Decreased libido
- o Depression
- o Dry hair
- o Dry, rough skin
- o Fatigue
- o Hair loss
- o Intolerance to Cold
- o Irritability
- o Memory loss
- o Muscle cramps and frequent muscle aches
- o Weakness
- o Weight gain or increased difficulty losing weight
- o Carpal Tunnel Syndrome

There may be signs of puffiness around the eyes, a slowing heart rate and a drop in body temperature as hypothyroidism becomes more severe. If left untreated, hypothyroidism may lead to heart failure and myxedema coma, a genuinely life threatening condition. Myxedema coma is usually triggered by severe illness, stress and surgery. This will require immediate treatment with thyroid hormone.

Hypothyroidism can strike anyone, at any age, and parents should be aware that even infants can develop the condition. Babies who suffer from hypothyroidism might not show any symptoms at all, but if they do, you will most likely see things like:

- Cold hands and feet
- Constipation
- Hoarse cry
- Little or no growth
- Extreme sleepiness
- Low muscle tone
- Persistent jaundice (yellowing of the skin and eyes)
- Poor feeding habits
- Puffy face
- Stomach bloating
- Swollen tongue

If your baby is showing any symptoms like these, you should contact your doctor for an appointment immediately. Bear in mind that these same symptoms can be caused by other medical conditions, as well, but even so, they bear checking out.

CAUSES & SYMPTOMS OF HASHIMOTO'S THYROIDITIS DISEASE

Hashimoto's disease is an autoimmune disorder, which means that your body basically creates antibodies that attack and do physical damage to your thyroid gland. This is the actual cause of Hashimoto's Thyroiditis disease, but it's still unclear as to what causes your body to create those antibodies which end up doing the damage.

While doctors are still unsure as to what causes your immune system to attack and damage your thyroid gland, many of them have come to believe that a virus or bacteria may be the trigger, as this is the case with many autoimmune disorders. Some doctors, however, tend to believe it may be the result of a genetic flaw.

While the question still remains up in the air as to the actual cause of the antibodies attacking your thyroid gland, there are certain contributory factors that may increase your risk of Hashimoto's thyroiditis disease:

Gender

Hashimoto's Thyroiditis Disease is 5 to 10 times more prevalent in women than in men.

Age

While Hashimoto's Thyroiditis disease may occur at any age it is much more common between the ages of 40 and 60.

Genetics

If members of your immediate family have a thyroid or other autoimmune disease, you are at a much higher risk of coming down with Hashimoto's Thyroiditis Disease.

Other autoimmune conditions

If you have another type of autoimmune conditions, such as type 1 diabetes, lupus or rheumatoid arthritis, your risk of having Hashimoto's disease is increased.

The actual symptoms of Hashimoto's Thyroiditis Disease are quite similar to the symptoms and signs of hypothyroidism, and can often be very subtle. As these conditions are not specific to Hashimoto's Thyroiditis Disease, they are often confused with other diseases or attributed to common aging symptoms. The symptoms usually will be much more obvious as the condition worsens

Common symptoms are:

- Aches and pains
- Cold intolerance
- Constipation
- Decreased concentration
- Depression
- Dry skin and hair
- Excessive fatigue and drowsiness

- Increased cholesterol
- Muscle cramps
- Carpal tunnel syndrome
- Swelling of the legs and extremities
- Weight gain

DIAGNOSIS & TREATMENT

If you are displaying more than a couple of the hypothyroidism symptoms described above, your doctor will almost certainly order blood tests to check on your hormone levels. These should include tests for proper levels of Thyroid-stimulating hormone (TSH) and for levels of T4 (thyroxine)

If your T4 levels are significantly lower than normal, then it is highly likely that you do suffer from hypothyroidism. However, it is possible that you may have increased TSH levels, while still displaying perfectly normal T4 levels. This is known as subclinical or mild hypothyroidism, and most doctors believe this to represent a very early stage of the full condition, so they'll want to confirm the diagnosis so that treatment can begin immediately.

If your blood test results are abnormal in any way related to the thyroid or its secretions, your doctor may order a thyroid ultrasound or scan to look for nodules or signs of inflammation.

An ultrasound is an imaging procedure that allows your doctor to visually examine the thyroid and parathyroid glands. A thyroid ultrasound lows the doctor to determine the actual size and shape of the thyroid, but it isn't able to give any information on how well the thyroid gland is functioning. An ultrasound may also be employed to check the parathyroid glands that are attached to the back edges of the thyroid.

During an ultrasound of the thyroid and parathyroid, a hand held device know as a transducer is moved gently back and forth over the neck, and the echos of the sound waves it emits are read by a computer in order to construct a visual image of the thyroid and parathyroid glands.

The reasons for performing this test can vary, and may include checking for lumps in the thyroid. The ultrasound technician or doctor can then determine whether any lumps found represent a solid nodule or a fluid-filled sac, or cyst.

The test is also used to determine whether the thyroid might be enlarged, a condition commonly know as a goiter. Goiter is an enlargement of the thyroid that is non cancerous. It is most commonly caused by an iodine deficiency in the diet, and may be a symptom of hyperthyroidism. In the US, iodized salt is commonly used and provides sufficient iodine that it is almost always considered part of hyperthyroidism. It can affect absolutely anyone regardless of age, gender, race or other factors, but they are most commonly seen in people who are beyond age of forty. Women are more susceptible to thyroid disorders, and risk factors include your medical history, the types of medications you have used, pregnancy, and exposure to radiation.

You may not show any symptoms if the goiter is not severe, or until it grows large enough to affect you. **Then you may see symptoms like:**

- Hoarseness
- Breathing and swallowing problems
- Coughing or wheezing
- Swelling or tightness of your neck

An ultrasound may be used to keep track of the size of the thyroid gland during treatment for a thyroid problem, and to watch for goiter to develop, or to guide placement of a needle if it becomes necessary to perform a thyroid biopsy.

When Hashimoto's Thyroiditis Disease is properly diagnosed, it can be easily treated with a thyroid hormone replacement treatment, but if it is left untreated it can often lead to some very severe complications.

When hypothyroidism is left untreated, it can worsen and bring on a number of serious and potentially life threatening complications. Making sure you can recognize the symptoms of hypothyroidism and asking your doctor to check for indications that you may have the condition can help you to avoid suffering any of the complications listed below.

Birth Defects

If you are pregnant while suffering an undetected thyroid disorder or one that has gone untreated, it's possible that your baby could have a significantly higher risk of suffering from birth defects than other children who are born to mothers in better health. Those who are born to mothers who have an untreated thyroid disorder could suffer from serious mental or physical development problems. This is due to the fact that thyroid hormones are necessary for the proper development of the brain during fetal growth.

In many cases, however, these kinds of problems can be treated after birth, allowing the child to regain healthy development. One of the tests commonly done in the newborn screening is a somewhat abbreviated test for thyroid issues.

Heart Problems

Even in its mildest forms, hypothyroidism can cause some serious heart problems. When the thyroid is not functioning as it should, it can cause an increased risk of heart disease due to the fact that it increases your levels of what doctors are now calling "bad" cholesterol. Excessive levels of this bad cholesterol can bring on hardening of the arteries, or atherosclerosis, which is likely to raise your risk of having a heart attack or a stroke.

Pericardial Effusion

Pericardial effusion is an abnormal and excessive accumulation of fluid around the heart, in the pericardial cavity. Since the space in the pericardial cavity is limited and fixed, any excess fluid buildup will cause significantly increased pressure in the cavity, and this pressure can affect your heart's ability to function normally and properly. If the pressure is great enough to have a serious effect on your heart function, it is known as cardiac tamponade, and is a life threatening condition.

Infertility

Whenever thyroid hormone levels fall below normal, they may affect ovulation and a woman's ability to conceive a child. Even after treatment for hypothyroidism with thyroid hormone supplement therapy, there is still the possibility that fertility may not return to normal, and conception may be difficult or impossible.

Mental Health Problems

Hypothyroidism can cause mental issues if it is left untreated for too long, and even mild hypothyroidism can bring on symptoms of depression. When there is no treatment, the symptoms of hypothyroidism will only grow worse, and this will have effects on your mental state, causing depression and other problems to intensify as a result. In addition, it has been shown in numerous studies that untreated hypothyroidism is directly related to a gradual loss of mental function.

Myxedema

Myxedema is term doctors use for extreme hypothyroidism, which is when the condition has continued for a long period of time without any treatment. Myxedema is quite rare, simply because of the low probability that someone would fail to realize that the worsening symptoms meant a serious problem and see a doctor for diagnosis and treatment.

However, this type of hypothyroidism is extremely life threatening, and can gradually slow your metabolism until you reach a point where you lapse into a coma. If you feel that you have any of the symptoms of myxedema, like unusually extreme fatigue or cold intolerance, contact a doctor immediately.

The trick to avoiding these potentially deadly complications that arise from untreated hypothyroidism is to recognize the symptoms of the disorder and get prompt medical attention. This condition is manageable as long as you are receiving the right treatment, and it actually need not interrupt or affect your daily life more than minimally.

All of these are symptoms and complications that you may experience with hypothyroidism, but remember that the condition itself is far too often only a symptom of Hashimoto's Thyroiditis, and so our focus is on that disease. We provide this additional information because it may aid you in determining whether you may be suffering from the disease and need to consult your doctor about proper diagnosis and treatment options. Let us now return to the main topic, and continue to provide you with the tools you need to combat or live with the disease.

At the onset of Hashimoto's Thyroiditis, most patients experience hyperthyroid, which is when the body produces too much of the thyroid hormone. This is caused by the leakage of thyroid hormone once the gland is damaged and being destroyed. Some people may experience a cycle of alternating hyperthyroidism and hypothyroidism, a condition known as hashitoxicosis.

Hashitoxicosis often causes doctors to misdiagnose Hashimoto's Thyroiditis, at least initially, as Graves' Disease, which causes the condition of Hyperthyroidism. This is why several lab tests should be taken, several days apart, in order to confirm any thyroid conditions or diseases.

Treatment Overview

Hypothyroidism is most easily treated through the use of thyroid hormone supplemental medications. The best and most effective thyroid hormone supplement is synthetic, and made in a laboratory. Once your treatment begins, you will need to maintain a regular schedule of visits to your doctor, in order to ensure you continue to receive the proper dosage of the medication.

With most patients, their symptoms begin to improve within a week after treatment is commenced, and all, or almost all of their symptoms are usually gone within just a few months. Babies and children who have hypothyroidism should always receive treatment, and as soon as possible after diagnosis. Older people, and those who suffer from poor health may not respond to the medicine as quickly as others.

If you have ever undergone radiation therapy and suffer from hypothyroidism, or if your thyroid gland has had to be taken out, you will most likely have to continue receiving treatment from now on. If your hypothyroidism is a result of Hashimoto's Thyroiditis, you might still have to have treatment from now on, but sometimes, thyroid function can return to normal on its own in Hashimoto's thyroiditis, although this is rare.

If your hypothyroidism was triggered by a serious illness or infection, then your thyroid function will most likely go back to normal when your recovery is complete or nearly complete. This is also the case with most forms of hypothyroidism caused by medications; when the medication is discontinued, the thyroid usually returns to normal function.

In cases of mild, subclinical hypothyroidism, treatment may not be required but should be watched for signs that your hypothyroidism is getting worse. You and your doctor will have to talk about the benefits, if any, of taking any type of medicines to treat mild hypothyroidism. The dosage would have to be watched carefully in cases of people who might also suffer from heart disease, since an excess of the medicine can increase risks of irregular heartbeats and chest pain.

Beginning Treatment

Your doctor will start your treatment with the thyroid medication levothyroxine. Take your medicine exactly as your doctor tells you to. You will need to have an additional blood test six-eight weeks after treatment begins, in order to be sure the dosage is right for you.

If you take enough of the medicine, you may continue to show symptoms of hypothyroidism, like gaining weight, feeling cold or sluggish, and constipation. Too much, in the other hand, can cause anxiety, difficulty in sleeping, and muscular tremors. People with heart disease usually start on a lower dosage of medication, which can be increased gradually as the doctor determines an increase to be safe or beneficial.

HOLISTIC TREATMENTS

Even over a hundred years after Hashimoto's Thyroiditis has been discovered and explained, doctors still are puzzled by many aspects of this disease. For example, as mentioned earlier, doctors are still not sure what causes your body to suddenly start attacking your thyroid gland. It may be something as simple as an allergic reaction to a certain type of food, or it could well be some other underlying condition that causes your body to see your thyroid gland as a threat to its own well-being.

Unfortunately, in today's medical practice, most doctors are too busy to actually try to find underlying causes for many conditions, and are too quick to simply prescribe this or that medication based on symptomatic data only, without further examining any other factors. This is one reason why it's a good idea to find a practitioner whose diagnostic techniques and treatments are holistic in nature.

Holistic, to put it in the simplest terms, means treating the whole person rather than simply focusing on a single condition or disease. In the case of Hashimoto's Thyroiditis, it means not simply treating the disease, but looking at the possible underlying causes of the disease and symptoms, and developing a treatment plan that will benefit the whole person.

It is imperative when managing Hashimoto's Thyroiditis, as well as other auto-immune disorders, that specific triggers be investigated that may cause auto-immune flair ups. One trigger that has been found to often be among the underlying causes of Hashimoto's Thyroiditis is gluten intolerance. Or to be more specific, gliaden sensitivity. Gliaden is the polypeptide found in gluten, and research has found that as much as 60% of Hashimoto's Thyroiditis patients will be gliaden sensitive.

Many experts and leaders in the field of Hashimoto's Thyroiditis research have theorized that gluten may be (at least in part) one of the underlying causes of Hashimoto's Thyroiditis, due to its molecular similarity with the Thyroid gland. The theory is that, once the gluten molecule enters the gut, the immune system will then look for other molecules that are similar to it, in order to produce antibodies to fight off something that it perceives as harmful. Because there are such similarities between the gluten molecule and that of the Thyroid Gland, it may well see the Thyroid as being comprised of these harmful molecules, automatically producing an antibody reaction to fight it.

While there are quite a few tests for gluten intolerance, they are not always accurate for a couple of reasons. One reason is that those people with weakened immune systems may not have enough anti-bodies in their body to show up on a standard blood or saliva test. Another reason is that these tests will only check for Alpha gliaden, which is only one variety of gliaden that a patient might be potentially allergic or sensitive to. A more thorough testing for all variations of gliaden may be much more beneficial when it comes to determining whether a patient does, indeed, have a gluten intolerance.

Another method of finding intolerance and allergies to foods is through an elimination diet, where all gluten cross-reactors are tested until they are determined to be either safe or harmful. While this method may take some time, it's probably the most effective in helping to treat patients and alleviate many underlying symptoms that may go completely undiscovered in the majority of patients suffering from Hashimoto's Thyroiditis and other thyroid and auto-immune related diseases and conditions.

With Hashimoto's Thyroiditis, there could be a host of other biological imbalances that may be affecting the production of thyroid hormones, such as liver functions, allergies and adrenal dysfunctions. In order to treat the conditions holistically, all of these should be taken into consideration before thyroid hormone replacement is considered.

While thyroid hormone replacements have been shown to be of great benefit to many patients, other means of treatment may be even more beneficial if an underlying cause for the disease can be found and treated, possibly even eliminating the need for a lifetime reliance on hormones.

The problem with a thyroid hormone replacement regiment is that, once you have started down that road, there is no turning back. This is due to the fact that synthetic hormone pills will cause your body to stop producing its own thyroid hormones. Keep in mind that sometimes patients are misdiagnosed with Hashimoto's Thyroiditis, where an underlying condition may not have been eliminated before patients have been prescribed hormonal replacement therapy (synthetic hormone pills).

This means that, in these instances, rare though they are, instead of helping to cure the patient, they may instead be helping to progress the disease of Hashimoto's Thyroiditis. If it is later found that those patients did not actually have Hashimoto's Thyroiditis to begin with, but some other underlying condition, those patients may not be able to be cured or treated properly, due to the body's inability to produce thyroid hormones on its own as a result of its forced dependence on the artificial hormone regimen.

This is why it's very important to find a practitioner of holistic medicine, who will take the time to go beyond standard tests before prescribing a synthetic drug that might actually cause more harm than good. Most holistic practitioners will be well acquainted with natural alternatives that aid in helping patients to overcome underlying symptoms so that they never need to rely on pharmaceutical medicines.

One of the most powerful natural treatments many practitioners have found in the treatment of Hashimoto's

Disease and other auto-immune disorders is Coconut Oil. This is due to the high amounts of various fatty acids found in Coconut Oil that contributes in helping to increase your body's metabolism. In addition, one of these fatty acids is Lauric acid, which is an essential fatty acid used by your body to help build and maintain a healthy immune system.

What this means is that different fatty acids in Coconut Oil positively affects the thyroid gland and helps in the production of thyroid hormones as well as affecting weight loss in most patients. Linoleic Acid, another fatty acid found in Coconut Oil, is a polyunsaturated fat that has been shown to help patients lose weight as well as promote the reduction of body fat.

Many experts have concluded that consuming 4 Tablespoons of Coconut oil per day may be enough to combat the effects of Hashimoto's Thyroiditis without the need for hormonal replacements. Not only is Coconut Oil helpful in combating Hashimoto's Thyroiditis, but it also aids your body in many other ways, such as weight loss, building your immune system and combating many other diseases and conditions.

Of course, you will need to talk to your doctor or medical practitioner before deciding on a more natural treatment plan. Your holistic doctor may be familiar with other natural remedies as well, such as essential oils and flower extracts that may help in conjunction with other treatments.

EATING RIGHT & LOSING WEIGHT

Many symptoms that occur with hypothyroidism can be offset by eating the right kinds of food and knowing what foods you should avoid. Many people are under the assumption that if you have hypothyroidism, then it is impossible to lose weight, but this is far from the case. While it's true that you won't lose weight at the same rate as you did before or at the same rate as someone else, with the proper diet and exercise, you can still lose weight.

First, you need to be realistic when making any weight loss goals, realizing that you may not be able to lose as much weight as you may want to, at least not to start off. After you have been on your thyroid hormone replacement therapy for a while, you will find it gets a little easier to lose weight, but still not as easy as someone who does not have Hashimoto's Thyroiditis.

You should not allow yourself to become discouraged if your weight doesn't come off as quickly as you like or if you have setbacks. However, by changing your diet and watching what you eat, you should be able to maintain a healthy weight, once the hormone therapy kicks in and your body is getting enough thyroid hormone to regulate itself.

You should concentrate on foods rich in Vitamin B as the B vitamins will help your body use your food to make energy. The foods that have the most vitamin B are usually high in protein. Brown rice, lentils and gluten free pasta are good choices, as are bananas, salmon (and most other fresh fish), baked potatoes, sweet potatoes, spinach, beef, poultry, shellfish, eggs, and some dairy products.

Fiber can provide bulk in your diet which will help to regulate your bowel movements, and is a necessity since constipation is one of the symptoms of Hashimoto's Thyroiditis. You should try to focus on those foods that are high in insoluble fiber and resistant starches. Soluble fiber and resistant starches are not digested, or not fully digested, by your body, which helps to aid you in keeping your bowel movements regular.

Bran is one food that is an excellent source of fiber; whether you are consuming oat bran, corn bran or rice bran, it's one of nature's very best sources of fiber.

You can also get your fiber from most beans, berries and whole grains. A "Whole Grain" is when the grain contains the entire seed of the plant, which is made up of the bran, germ and endosperm. When they "refine" grains, they remove the germ and bran, which removes the fiber, protein and many other key nutrients. White rice, for example, is refined rice, while brown rice still has the germ and bran layer. Avoid any refined grains, and as we'll see in a bit, it's best to avoid grains whenever possible.

Another good source of fiber and vitamins is leafy green vegetables, or "Greens", such as Lettuce, Cabbage,

Turnip Greens, Mustard Greens, Collard Greens and Spinach.

Do be sure to increase your water intake, as your body will require more water in order to move the insoluble fiber through your colon. Besides, proper hydration is essential to almost every part of your body, and not hydrating yourself as needed can lead to many other problems, such as lethargy, muscle spasms and cramps and more.

One of the great things about eating foods high in fiber is that you will feel full faster. This factor will help to curb your appetite and allow you to eat less and lose weight more easily.

One of the side effects of hypothyroidism is that you feel tired and lack energy. Many people find themselves relying on high calorie foods to combat the feelings of fatigue, which, of course, leads to greater weight gain. You do need to focus on complex carbs in order to provide your body with the necessary energy, but you need to be sure to limit your intake of carbs and fiber, and to eat the high fiber, high carb foods such as fruits, brown rice and beans early in the day, when your body requires more energy. You should eat more leafy green vegetables and lean proteins later in the day, or as your last meal of the day.

Since gluten intolerance is known to be related to Hashimoto's Thyroiditis Disease, one thing you must consider is the elimination of gluten, and especially wheat gluten, from your diet. This will mean a rather complete lifestyle change, since wheat products permeate almost everything found in the local grocery store. Let's look at this in greater depth.

The Problem With Wheat

Wheat permeates so much of our diets today, in so many ways, that the very thought of trying to avoid consuming it can be overwhelming. However, the relationship between gluten and thyroid problems is so well documented that it is a necessity if you intend to live a normal, healthy life with Hashimoto's Thyroiditis or hypothyroidism. For this reason, we will give you a number of reasons for this lifestyle change, but first, let's look at why it's even necessary to discuss it.

For thousands of years, man has consumed wheat in one form or another. It has been used as bread, stuffing in birds and meats, thickener for soups and stews and gravies, as crackers and cookies and cakes and just about every other way you can imagine. If you look back over history, it's certain that you'll find wheat in one of its forms scattered over the centuries. Moses and the Israelites ate wheat in the forms of unleavened bread; Jesus ate bread with his disciples; biscuits and crackers traveled across the ocean with Christopher Columbus, and went with the Spaniards and the British and everyone else who traveled throughout the world.

And then came the industrial revolution. Machines were invented that could harvest wheat faster than men could do, and shipping became so much more efficient than the horse and wagon that wheat products could be made in one place and sold in another. As progress evolved in our modern world, the demand for wheat went higher every day.

Enter the geneticist. By crossbreeding different strains of wheat, new varieties were created that grew faster, grew bigger grains, grew more grains per stalk. More foods could be made from wheat products, because the supply was up; before long, we were seeing whole new kinds of cereals, breads, snacks, pastas and many other things made from wheat.

The science, however, that made these new kinds of wheat didn't bother to loo closely at the less visible changes that were occurring in the wheat they were producing. The new strains contained far more gluten and opioid peptides than man had ever consumed before, and these components of modern wheat can do significant harm to the human body.

Gluten

Gluten can cause inflammation of the gut in more than three quarters of the people in our modern world, and at least another third will develop antibodies against gluten proteins. What isn't as obvious is that virtually all of the world's people could, and likely will, develop antibodies against gluten. There's the possibility that this could be good news, because when your body doesn't have a reaction to gluten right off the bat, the gluten proteins can get into the blood stream. This is especially true if you have what's known as a "leaky gut," and can easily trigger immune system reactions at some other point in the body.

Since gliadin, the gluten protein that causes the most problems, is very similar in molecular structure to the molecules of tissues in organs like the thyroid or the pancreas, anti-gliadin antibodies will eventually start to attack those organs, ultimately causing autoimmune diseases like hypothyroidism or diabetes type 1.

Gluten based inflammation of the intestines causes the cells there to die off, as well as causing those cells to become oxidized. This is what causes a leaky gut, which can allow bacteria and other things to migrate into the bloodstream, and this leads to the autoimmune attacks on various organs. A leaky gut can also mean that food cannot be properly digested, meaning that nutrients are not fully absorbed. This leads to nutritional deficiencies that are dangerous in their own right.

Anti-gluten antibodies have also been found to attack tissues in the heart, leading to damages that causes heart disease. These effects can cause things like enlargement of the heart muscle, irregular heartbeat and chest pain, as well as other effects that can go unnoticed until they become severe.

Lastly, we should tell you that gluten appears to be capable of causing, or at least exacerbating, some cancers. All of the data is not in yet, and studies are still ongoing into this concern.

WGA (wheat germ agglutinin)

Like gluten, WGA causes irritation, inflammation and premature cell death in the intestine and is likely to lead to a leaky gut condition, with all the problems that usually follow along with it. It breaks down the cells of the mucus membrane in the intestine, leading ultimately to bacterial overgrowth and a significant number of other digestive problems such as GERD and ulcers.

Leptin begins circulating throughout the body and in the brain, where it can have effects that are similar to those of insulin. This means that it is a probable cause or enabler of obesity, because leptin and insulin are the most critical hormones the body needs to regulate properly in order to keep the body at a normal weight vs. energy balance.

WGA, when combined with another, unidentified factor in wheat, causes vitamin D levels to fall rapidly, which will lead to a vitamin D deficiency. This brings along its own issues, like porosity and weakening of the bones, a less effective immune system and susceptibility to many different contagious diseases and bacterial infections.

Opioid peptides

They're referred to as "opioids" because their molecular structure is very similar to certain derivatives of opium. The particular opioid peptides that are commonly found in modern wheat can actually cause addiction to wheat in many people. It is quite possible for someone to suffer through genuine withdrawal symptoms when wheat is completely removed from the diet.

These peptides are also thought to be associated with some types of schizophrenia, and may be a root cause or promoter of the condition. Schizophrenic patients have actually seen their symptoms fade away when they eliminate wheat products from their own diets.

The fact is, we humans are simply not designed to eat and digest wheat. The destructive effects of its gluten proteins are some of the most devastating out of all the foods we eat. Unfortunately, wheat and its thousands of products make up a multi-billion dollar a year industry, and even the medical community is involved. Doctors, many of whom truly do know better, are constantly recommending "whole wheat," "whole grain breads" and other wheat containing diets that contribute to the rise of such things as obesity, type II diabetes, celiac disease and more, and there is evidence to suggest that it is related to the rise in autism cases over the past fifty years. There are so many health problems that would almost certainly not exist except for our modern extreme consumption of wheat and wheat products. Those who eliminate wheat and other glutens from their diets often see improvement in their health conditions almost immediately.

Granted, most people can indulge in some wheat products occasionally without suffering major negative effects, but wheat and other grains should probably be completely avoided, especially among those who have any type of autoimmune disease or inflammatory condition. This includes conditions such as arthritis, lupus and, of course, Hashimoto's Thyroiditis and hypothyroidism.

The Milk Dilemma

Along with the almost universal problem of gluten intolerance, estimates of those who are unable to digest cow's milk and many of its products range from thirty to a whopping seventy percent, depending on which study you choose to accept as most credible. Even if you opt for the one with the lowest numbers, though, what you can't fail to acknowledge is that the facts suggest that doctors who push milk as being good for you are doing nothing but promoting the multi-billion dollar dairy industry, and government agencies that insist "Milk, it does a body good," are doing so not for the health and well being of Americans, but for the dairy dollars that lobbyists throw around like water on a garden.

Even for those who are not allergic or sensitive to milk and milk products, there remains the fact that the calcium in cow's milk—the part of the milk that doctors and governments insist is necessary—can be only partially absorbed without supplementing the diet with magnesium. In addition, the pasteurization process makes most of that calcium insoluble (and eliminates all of its vitamin C), and therefore worthless to the human body, in any event. Since pasteurized milk is the only milk that you can find in any grocery store, when you talk about milk as a healthy addition to a diet, you're blowing smoke; there's no evidence to support it, and the only agency who actually says it's good for you is the National Dairy Council in a shameless self-promotional PR campaign.

For one thing, and please check this for yourself, if you live in the United States of America, then almost every cow used in the production of milk for pasteurization and mass marketing in American grocery stores is being treated with Monsanto's genetically engineered Bovine Growth Hormone, which is known to cause cancer and other diseases, especially in children. Are you willing to risk your children's health for the convenience of being able to grab a gallon of milk at the bog box grocer?

Frankly, you can get far more calcium, and actually absorb and benefit from it, by having a serving of leafy greens, such as spinach, eating almonds or sesame seeds, dry beans, wild salmon or sardines or even okra! And ignore the labels on foods that claim to be calcium fortified; they're worthless, since the things they're added to have even worse health effects than a calcium deficiency.

One of the most common alternatives to drinking pasteurized, mass produced, cancer causing cow's milk is to switch to goat's milk. Granted, it can be more expensive, but it can be easily digested by almost everyone, it has more calcium that can actually be absorbed by humans, and it contains more of the essential fatty acids that our bodies need.

Most people who try goat's milk find that it tastes better than cow's milk, as well. It can be used in cooking in place of cow's milk, and often gives foods made with it a more enjoyable flavor than they had before. It's great on cereals, and fine just by itself. It can be used to make cheeses, creams, ice cream and just about anything else that cow's milk can be used for.

The only thing it won't do is make you feel sick or cause you health problems (okay, unless you are on of the estimated one to one and a half percent who have an actual milk allergy, and not a simple lactose intolerance—very rare). If you're going to truly eat healthy, getting rid of the milk that is almost certainly causing you problems is important.

Many people with Hashimoto's thyroiditis may suffer from an intolerance to milk proteins, egg proteins or soy proteins. Most of such cases go undiscovered, so that as people continue to consume these items, they are causing significant damage to their intestines and costing themselves vital nutrients. That may come as a surprise, but it's been found that even a great number of people who are overweight turn out to be completely malnourished and suffering from nutrient deficiency due to the foods they eat.

Actual food allergies are controlled by a part of the immune system called IgE. Their effects become apparent almost immediately when an allergen is consumed, which is why doctors and allergists often refer them as true allergies. However, that isn't an accurate name, and implies that only IgE allergies exist. In fact, there are reactions that are controlled by other parts of the immune system that are equally damaging and just as real. In fact, there are at least two more segments of the immune system that control reactions to foods, and they are the IgA and IgG segments.

For lack of a more fitting name, IgA and IgG type sensitivities are both known commonly as food intolerances or food sensitivities. In spite of this unfortunate use of inaccurate names, they act quite differently in their methods and abilities to cause harm to the human body.

IgA Reactions

IgA intolerances are more severe reactions and tend to work mostly in the intestines. They are abnormal responses of the intestines and intestinal walls to certain foods, and this is especially true in genetically predisposed patients. These problems may show up in early childhood, or years later, but they'll make themselves known when they do, by causing irritation and inflammation of the intestines every time the culprit food is eaten. This causes cumulative damage to the intestines, until they are no longer even able to absorb nutrients. This increases the risk of cancer, accelerate aging and autoimmune diseases such as hypothyroidism because it increases intestinal permeability—leaky gut.

These food intolerances may not display any symptoms at all, or they may show any or all of the following: constipation, diarrhea, loose stools, acid reflux, malnutrition and leaky gut syndrome.

The most common of these reactions is known as celiac disease, and it is a rather serious intolerance to gluten.

However, dairy protein intolerances are also very, very common in people who suffer from Hashimoto's Thyroiditis. These particular IgA intolerances have no specific name and are quite often mistaken for other, less serious food reactions.

We should mention here that lactose intolerance and dairy protein intolerance are two entirely different kinds of problems. Lactose is a kind of sugar, and our ability to digest it is dependent on our bodies having a natural enzyme called lactase, or possessing intestinal bacteria which can digest the sugar. Lactose intolerance can cause diarrhea, bloating and other issues, but normally will not produce intestinal tissue damage or inflammation.

What it all boils down to is that, if you suffer from Hashimoto's Thyroiditis but a gluten free diet doesn't seem to be making as big a difference as you expected, then it's time to look more closely and think about other foods that keeping your body from healing as it should. Milk proteins may well be another source of trouble.

The Myth of Soy

Soy has gained a reputation in recent years of being a health food, with stories about how, while it is a plant protein, it matches eggs and milk in terms of actual protein value and amino acid content. Unfortunately, nothing could be further from the truth. Let's take a look at this misconception in the mind of the public came to be.

Some years ago, tropical oils like palm and coconut oil were regularly used in the production of many American foods. Obviously, however, these oils are not domestic to the United States of America; except for Hawaii and possibly some parts of Florida, our climate just isn't tropical enough.

But food production costs money, and the more it costs, the lower the profits the food industry makes. With such financial incentives, the entire industry worked to devise a way to move away from tropical oils, and onto something that was more locally available and less expensive. The result was a plan to make tropical oils appear unhealthy and undesirable, so that they could be easily replaced with domestically grown oils like corn and soy.

The entire plan to paint soy as the healthy alternative to these supposedly unhealthy oils was an unqualified success, so what you're about to learn may disappoint and even upset some people. In particular, vegetarians and vegans have come to regard soy as one of their primary sources of protein.

However, there have been many studies on the health benefits of soy, and the general consensus is that unless the soy you're using is fermented, you may very well be putting your own health at risk. Soy, in fact, contains numerous unhealthy compounds that can cause many problems with your health, like:

Goitrogens—Goitrogens are found in all types of unfermented soy, regardless of whether it's organic or not. These are compounds that can prevent the production of thyroid hormones and interfere with the metabolism of iodine, and thus cause interference with your body's natural thyroid function. One of the most common sources of soy protein that people consume is through soy milk. Many people use it as an alternative to dairy products, or even as a simple beverage, just as cow's milk is used. Soy milk is a major contributor to thyroid problems or hypothyroidism in women in the United States, so if you're a woman who's dealing with poor thyroid function and you're using soy milk, there's a really big chance that you should stop drinking it immediately.

Isoflavones: genistein and daidzein—Isoflavones are a form of phytoestrogen, and this is a plant compound that is very similar to human estrogen. For this reason, some doctors actually suggest using soy products almost as a medicine, to deal with the symptoms of menopause. Any evidence in favor of this is extremely controversial, and there is actually very little chance that it works. In general, most people today are exposed to too much estrogen and already have a much lower testosterone level than they should, so it can be very critical to limit your exposure to these feminizing compounds.

Even more concerning, there is mounting evidence that these same compounds may promote breast cancer, cause infertility and disrupt normal endocrine function, which should without any doubt be a significant concern to everyone. Drinking just two glasses of soy milk each day for only one month gives your body enough of these phytonutrients to disrupt your menstrual cycle, and even though the FDA regulates all other estrogen-containing products, they have been amazingly silent about soy.

Phytic acid—Phytates attach themselves to ions of metal, which prevents your body from absorbing certain necessary minerals. These include magnesium, calcium, iron, and zinc, which are all things that you need to keep your body operating at its optimum levels. This is especially troublesome for vegans and vegetarians, since eating meat actually reduces their mineral-blocking effects.

There are actually times when this can be helpful, especially in women who are postmenopausal, and in the majority of men, because we have a tendency to have high iron levels. Iron is a very powerful oxidant and can cause significant physical stress. Phytic acid, however, does not just reduce iron absorption; it interferes with the absorption of all minerals. This is very important, since many people already deal with mineral deficiencies from an improper diet.

Soybeans have just about the highest phytate levels of any plant food, and those in soy are extremely resistant to the usual ways of reducing phytates, like long, slow cooking. In general, only a fairly long fermentation period will reduce the phytate content enough to matter.

Anti-nutrients—Soy contains other compounds known as anti-nutrients. These are things like protease inhibitors, saponins, oxalates, andsoyatoxin. Some of these can interfere with the enzymes your body requires in order to digest proteins. While a little bit of these would probably not cause a problem, many Americans are now eating an extremely high amount of soy and soy products, so the risk is very real.

Hemagglutinin—Hemagglutinin is a clotting agent that causes your red blood cells to clump together. Clumped, clotted cells are not able to absorb and transport oxygen to your body's tissues properly.

These dietary issues may seem overwhelming to you, especially since you've heard for so many years that these things were good for you. Eliminating them from your diet will mean a major lifestyle change, but there are many online resources that will confirm for you the validity of this information. We urge you to check it out for yourself.

EVERYDAY CHOICES (CHANGING YOUR LIFESTYLE IN OTHER WAYS, ONE CHOICE AT A TIME)

Hypothyroidism is a lifetime condition and, therefore, you will have to deal with it for the rest of your life. You can live a healthy normal life, but you will have to make some changes, particularly if you currently aren't making the healthiest choices.

Every choice you make is a step forward or a step backward to a healthy lifestyle. For instance, when you wake up in the morning, you can choose to eat a healthy breakfast consisting of gluten free foods, fresh fruits and goat's milk, or you can eat a donut and drink some coffee laden with sugar. Of course the first choice is the best choice, but in our busy lives, sometimes it's easier to grab a quick snack than take the time to eat right and take care of our bodies.

Another choice you may make, after eating your rice bran muffin with fresh squeezed orange juice, is to either drive to work, or walk. Walking is one of the most health benefiting activities you can engage in, but in today's society, it's almost unheard of to actually walk to work and leave your car in the driveway, even if work is only one or two miles away. If your job is too far to walk to, you might choose to park a mile or so away from your office or plant and walk the rest of the way. At the very least, you should always park at the outer edge of the parking lot; the two hundred yards or so you'll walk to get into the store or building is still exercise, and good for you.

At home, you can make a choice of whether you would like to lounge on the couch, take it easy, eat some popcorn and watch the idiot tube, or you can take the opportunity to do some exercises, get out for a walk (or a jog if you are so inclined) or to find some other activity that can give your body and mind a good workout.

Of course, you will also want to make time to relax, perhaps to meditate or just enjoy a good book, but each choice you make should be a conscious decision for your better health. Even if you aren't suffering from Hashimoto's Thyroiditis yourself, changing your lifestyle is in your best interest. However, with any kind of thyroid condition, it's imperative to take a look at each choice in your life and to make the decisions that have the best impact on your health and well being.

You should also remember, it's not really practical to believe you can change your whole lifestyle at one time. Changing your lifestyle one choice at a time is a much more practical approach. For instance, start with your diet. Instead of loading up on those foods that contain refined sugars and processed foods, on your next shopping trip stock up on fresh fruits, green leafy vegetables, proteins and bran foods; in other words, shop healthy, paying close attention to fiber and vitamins, and staying away from those simple carbs, i.e., sugars.

Once you have changed your eating lifestyle and have become accustomed to eating healthy, then you might change your exercise routine, adding in such things as walking, jogging, calisthenics, yoga (which is great for body and mind) and other activities that will help your body utilize the carbohydrates by turning them into energy instead of storing them as fat.

You could start by simply rising an hour earlier in the morning and going out for a brisk walk before breakfast. Once you get into a habit of doing this, you'll find that your body actually craves this morning routine. You'll feel better throughout the day, and you will find you have more energy and more vitality. It's a simple step which will reap great rewards.

In essence, you should focus on your health and well being and make it a habit to choose those things that will improve them, even (and especially) when you feel fatigued and simply don't have the energy. This doesn't mean your lifestyle is ONLY about exercise and eating healthy foods, but it should always be geared toward keeping your body and mind as healthy as you possibly can. It's okay to splurge every once in a while; go ahead and eat that piece of cheesecake, or take it easy and watch your favorite show once in a while, but don't make it your lifestyle—make it an exception, perhaps even a reward when you've been doing well.

LOOKING AT THE WHOLE PICTURE

If you have been diagnosed with Hashimoto's Thyroiditis, it doesn't have to be a life sentence of poor health and increased weight gain. It could be a wake up call for you that it's time to look at the whole picture of your current lifestyle, it may be a call to action on your part. If you look at it this way, you may find that, as awful as it seems on the surface, it could be a good thing this has happened to you.

I know it sounds ridiculous to say it may be a good thing, especially on the surface, but if you think about it, there may be a reason why your body is turning against you and this horrible disease may be just what you needed to realize that you haven't been treating your body right in the first place. This disease is treatable and it really doesn't have to bring you down, but you have to make a conscious decision to change your lifestyle, to start eating healthier and to start exercising.

There are many diseases and conditions related to lack of exercise and poor eating habits, and if you are one of those who lead a sedentary lifestyle and make poor dietary choices, you will eventually end up with some condition, whether it be Hashimoto's Thyroiditis, High Cholesterol, Heart Disease or a plethora of other possible conditions and diseases. To be blunt, if you don't treat your body right, your body will eventually break down and eventually you will die.

However, this needn't be the case. You can live a long, happy and healthy life, even with Hashimoto's Thyroiditis, if you take your medication regularly, eat healthy and make those lifestyle changes that impact your overall well being. It's up to you, though, to make those changes. No amount of medications will make your body healthy, nor will vitamin supplements make up for a healthy diet.

Regardless of your condition, your age, race or locality, regardless of your past or your heredity, you can make the decision to live healthier, to eat right and to get up off the couch and get active, walk more, start a garden, take an aerobics class, learn some yoga techniques. Do it for yourself, starting today.

Today is the first day of the rest of your life. Do you want to continue down the same road you were on, or do you want to take control of your health and your well being? Do you know that a healthy body is a healthy mind? What this means is when you start concentrating on keeping your body healthy, you will feel better about yourself, you will be happier and you will be able to focus on the important things in life.

When you start taking control of your life, by eating right and exercising right, your whole life will change. You will find yourself doing things you never did before, you will find yourself enjoying things you never thought you would enjoy, going places you had never thought about going and you will find yourself looking forward to each new day's challenges. Instead of avoiding life, you will find yourself embracing it.

Hashimoto's Thyroiditis might seem an awful disease, but once you accept that it is more than likely your lifestyle choices that have brought you to this point, and you make a conscious effort to change your life and those choices, then you may one day look back and see that this disease was the best thing that ever happened to you, as it made you examine who you are and how you are treating yourself, and thereby forced you to make those changes necessary to improve your health and your life.

28778732R00032

Made in the USA
Middletown, DE
27 January 2016